THE
Skin Care
BOOK

The Skin Care Book
Kathlyn Quatrochi

The information in this book should not be used as a substitute for advice from a qualified health-care practitioner.
Some ingredients may cause allergic reactions in susceptible individuals, and others may not be right to use for particular skin conditions.

Photography, Joe Coca

Text copyright 1997, Kathlyn Quatrochi
Photography copyright 1997, Joe Coca and Interweave Press

 Interweave Press, Inc.
201 East Fourth Street
Loveland, Colorado 80537
USA

Printed in Hong Kong by Sing Cheong

Library of Congress Cataloging-in-Publication Data
    Quatrochi, Kathlyn, 1954–
        The Skin care book : simple herbal recipes / Kathlyn Quatrochi.
            p.   cm.
        Includes bibliographical references and index.
        ISBN 1-883010-24-1
        1. Skin—Care and hygiene.   2. Herbal cosmetics.   I. Title.
    RL87.Q38   1997
    646.7'26—dc21   96-29747
                                                                  CIP

First Printing: IWP10M:197:CC

THE
Skin Care
BOOK
SIMPLE HERBAL RECIPES

KATHLYN QUATROCHI

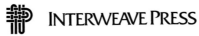 INTERWEAVE PRESS

To my clients, who enthusiastically allowed me to conduct

research on their faces over the past twenty years.

Their beautiful and healthy complexions stand out in a crowd

and continue to be my best advertising. I thank you.

ACKNOWLEDGEMENTS

For technical confirmations, inspiration, and encouragement,
my sincere thanks go to Nancy Anderson, M.D., George Dillinger,
M.D., James Munson, M.D., Laurel Munson, M.D.,
Joseph Quatrochi, and Norman Stanley. For patience, support,
and organization, thanks go to my editor Judith Durant.

PREFACE

Little did my family or I know that day many years ago when I got a huge splinter in my toe that I had started my walk along a path of botanical remedies. Nor could we have imagined where that path would lead: to my becoming a Master Herbalist, a Doctor of Naturopathy, and to my teaching about, using, selling, prescribing, and writing about natural treatments. The potato-and-bacon poultice Mom used on my toe didn't impress the emergency room doctor until he saw that it drew out the splinter. I didn't give it much thought at the time—I was used to using mud on stings, mustard plasters for chest colds, aloe on burns, and comfrey on cuts. These and many others were common cures at our home in Riverside, California.

The salubrious education I received from three generations of my family remains with me. Through my being a patient and then a student of George Dillinger, M.D., I learned that the doctorings my forebears had taught me were not just "home cures". And the scientific evidence I studied for my doctorate degree confirmed that herbs and many other natural substances can impact the health and well-being of the human body.

As a seventeen-year-old, I imagined I would grow up to be an environmental scientist working to end the pollution of our planet. I now find myself treating the pollution of our bodies. The path I embarked upon so many years ago has lead to a remarkably gratifying business through which I can share my knowledge by teaching classes and providing treatments. Now I can offer my insights to you, and hope you will use these herbal recipes to enhance your own inner beauty.

TABLE OF CONTENTS

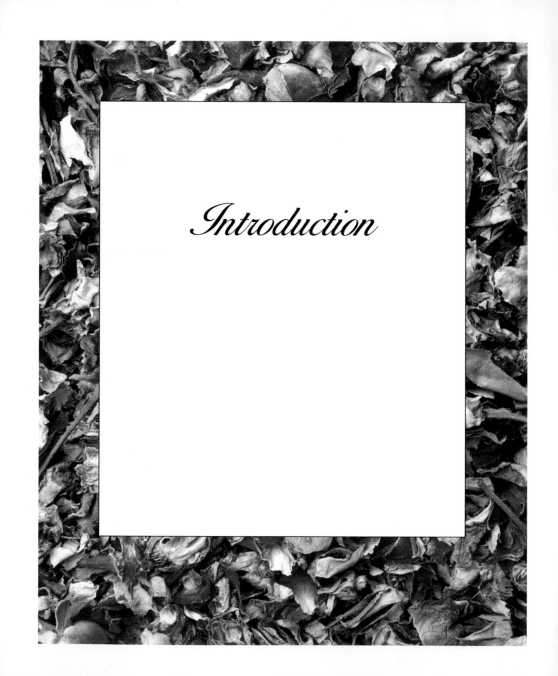

Introduction

For so many people everywhere—and especially here in Southern California, where I live—a ruthless pursuit of beauty is under way. Television and movies dangle ideals and unreasonable expectations in front of us. Cosmetic companies market their products aggressively and fan the fires of our vanity with promises that no little bottle could ever deliver. For some people, beauty has no price, and the quest becomes a series of fad diets, obsessive exercise, even cosmetic surgery. And the beauty chase inevitably disappoints us.

When I started in the skin-care business in Southern California twenty-five years ago, selling commercial cosmetics out of my home, health and beauty were separate, divergent goals. People were still greasing up with baby oil and lying in the sun to get the darkest tan possible—without a thought to skin cancer. There was emphasis on using makeup as camouflage. In the 1970s, society looked for chemical magic. In addition to eye makeup, lipstick, and rouge, the industry sold us face cream, eye cream, day cream, night cream, throat cream, and more. We really wanted to believe that we needed and would benefit from all those concoctions. The bottles were beautiful, the products smelled fabulous, and they made us feel better about ourselves. And when a particular product didn't live up to its advertising, we didn't hold the manufacturer accountable—

we just tried another brand of promises we'd seen advertised. The cycle has continued endlessly, and today cosmetics is a multibillion-dollar industry.

My wakeup call came in the form of a problem my little sister experienced at the age of thirteen. She started losing her hair, and doctors couldn't explain her bald patches. After a long ordeal, we finally traced her condition to the use of a common cosmetic that contained large amounts of a heavy metal. She had heavy-metal poisoning, yet because metal is a natural substance, a cosmetic containing it can boast "natural" on its label. It was eye-opening for me to learn that there was then and still is no regulating authority for the cosmetic industry.

I no longer felt at ease using commercial products on my skin. I wanted a more thorough knowledge and understanding of the ingredients that went into skin-care products. I began researching the topic, reading textbooks, talking to chemists, medical doctors, dermatologists, and learning as much as I could about the field of cosmetics. I was surprised to learn that many cosmetics relied on poisonous substances to attain results. Arsenic, for example, induces mild swelling and redness of the skin, causing a reduction of wrinkles and large pores and producing a rosy glow. Arsenic is also a "natural" substance, yet it can accumulate in the body and cause ill effects such as liver disease, depression, a depressed immune system, hair loss, and even death—effects that you may never suspect to have originated from your cosmetics.

I also learned a lot about how the skin functions, from the inside out and the outside in. The more I learned, the more convinced I became that for skin to work as nature intended and to be beautiful as a result, commercial cosmetics were not the answer. Perhaps my greatest revelation was the realization that the home remedies from Mom and Grandma that I been raised on—such as mustard plasters, potato poultices, oatmeal masques, vinegar hair rinses, herbal facials, and many other formulas—worked just fine and were far kinder to my skin than the expensive cosmetics I had been using.

I made a commitment to develop my own skin-care products, and over the years, I've discovered many treatments and formulas that really work! Skin care has become both a passion and a business for me, and I can see the results of these safe, natural products in my clients' faces. Glowing complexions of people who have used my products for twenty years now are the beautiful proof of their effectiveness. I feel good about skin care that doesn't come at the cost of health and integrity and without much strain on pocketbooks—and about passing on this knowledge to other people.

In this book, I'll show you how to take charge of your own skin care. In your own kitchen, using ingredients from your garden, cupboards, grocery store, and corner pharmacy, you can make skin treatments that you can rely on, feel comfortable using, and see the results of when you look in the mirror. I'll show you how to be beautiful.

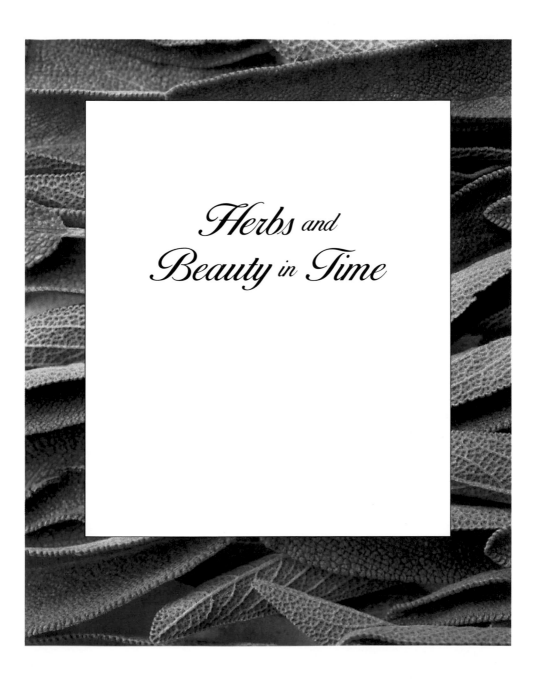

Herbs and
Beauty in *Time*

The use of herbs and other natural substances in the pursuit of beautiful skin goes back at least to 5000 B.C., when the Egyptians, and then the Greeks, Chinese, and Romans, used oils and herbs to make bath products and perfumes. Herbs and minerals such as chamomile and henna were then, and are still, used to make eye makeup and dyes for hair and nails. We have all heard of Cleopatra's milk baths, and have seen her cobalt eyeliner depicted in historical pictures and anthropological discoveries. Egyptian hieroglyphics from the Nile Valley depict bodies painted for beauty and religious ceremony. Soaps were used as far back as 2200 B.C. Later, herbs were combined with them for beauty purposes. Special herb teas were consumed to "feed" a beautiful complexion.

Native Americans exploited both the healing and beautifying power of herbs. They made beautifully colored face paints from herbs and clays; they also recognized the saponic nature of herbs such as yucca, and used them for washing. American Indians also used sage and mint decoctions topically for acne treatment. Squaw vine made into an ointment was a blessing for nursing mothers with sore nipples. Lobelia, also known as Indian Tobacco, was used to relieve painful skin infections and ringworm.

Some of our own mothers and grandmothers, and indeed, some of us, have used henna to tint hair, oatmeal masques to purify skin, witch hazel as an astringent, and mentholated salves for soft lips. My great grandfather used an herbal lotion of lanolin and comfrey to keep his "farmer's hands" from chapping.

In the recent past, people became excited by new synthetic discoveries. However, as we become more environmentally conscious, we wonder about the impact of synthetics on our world and question what is safe and what is not. Looking at old-fashioned remedies, we find opportunity to acknowledge the chemical values of herbs and other natural substances. For example, lavender and witch hazel help to heal wounds because they contain chemical properties that are astringent, antibiotic, and that encourage cell reproduction. Many other herbs naturally contain constituents that promote health and healing and can ultimately lead to your best complexion.

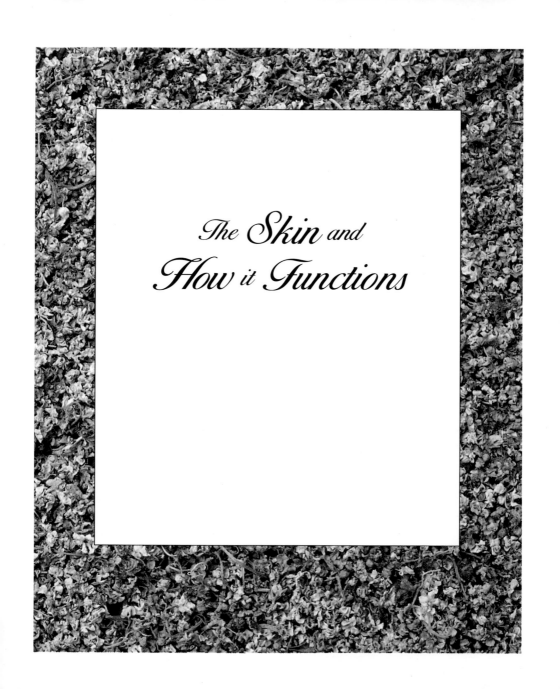

The Skin and
How it Functions

Your skin is the largest organ of your body; it is alive and ever-changing. It constantly generates new cells during a renewing cycle that takes about twenty-six days. The skin protects all the other organs by covering them and maintaining body temperature, and it continually cleanses the whole system by releasing the impurities deposited by capillaries through perspiration and sebum (oil).

The skin varies in thickness from 1/32 to 1/3 of an inch. It consists of two distinct layers, the epidermis and the dermis. Each of these layers has many other layers.

The epidermis is the outer layer, and is a mass of dead cells that are continually being rubbed off and replaced by newly dead cells as they rise from the lower layer.

The dermis is the lower layer, and it contains the tissues and glands that produce new skin, nails, hair, protein fiber, and collagen, which provides tissue support and elasticity. The other important elements of the dermis are the sebaceous (oil) glands, and sweat (moisture) glands, more than three million in all. These glands produce the essential fluids that make a healthy complexion. These fluids have lipophilic (fat) and hydrophilic (water) properties, and we recognize them as oily secretions and perspiration. The excretions of oil and water create a film, called the acid mantle, on the surface of the skin; this film helps to protect us from the elements and disease. The pH of this film is slightly acidic and supports healthy or good bacteria while warding off or killing harmful ones. (The pH scale is the measure of acidity and alkalinity. The scale is from 0 to 14, with 0 being most acid and 14 being most alkaline.) Healthy skin should have a pH of between 4.5 and 5.5, and some topical applications can help restore the acid mantle to a sound pH level.

However, no topical application of any product or concoction can make up for the impact of poor diet, lack of rest, lack of exercise, poor breathing, or environmental factors such as smog, polluted water, hydrocarbons, and fluorescent lighting on the skin. At the time of this writing, the nutritional fad is low-fat, high-complex carbohydrate. There are many companies and diet centers that will help you maintain this sort of diet. Many people believe that if reducing fat is good, then the less you have, the better! But how does a great reduction of fat intake affect your skin?

Fat, water, and protein intake all affect the function and appearance of the skin. A drastic reduction of any of these substances may change your physique, but some of my clients who have practiced these diets have had their skin age about twenty years in appearance! Fat supports the skin by retaining water, thereby keeping it firm and elastic. Once lost, it is almost impossible to rebuild skin elasticity to its ultimate condition. We can regain some, but it may take years.

Even well-fed skin is challenged by our environment and the process of aging or oxidation. So just what can we do to create, maintain, and protect our complexions? We know that our skin needs a balance of both oil and water to provide a smooth surface. We need proteins such as collagen for support, and skin-surface pH should be slightly acidic to keep harmful fungi and viruses that can cause skin damage as well as internal disease in check.

This basic knowledge helps us to begin to analyze our own skin needs. I have seen clients who say their skin is dry, only to find that it is quite oily. Dead cells are held onto the skin by oils; these cells do not fall off easily, so the skin appears dry.

I am not fond of labeling anyone's skin "oily" or "dry". These are temporary conditions which can be corrected. The skin becomes unbalanced in reaction to inappropriate diet, environment, topical care, and even stress. For example, stress depletes vitamins C and E. Vitamin C aids the production of collagen; too little collagen promotes wrinkles. Vitamin E contains essential fatty acids and is an antioxidant which helps slow the aging process.

Fortunately, some topical skin care can help to support your body's natural abilities to keep skin healthy and glowing.

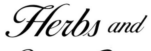

Herbs and
Skin Care

Herbs and other natural substances can affect the skin in many ways. In addition to their hydrophilic and lipophilic properties and their ability to impart acid or alkaline conditions to the skin surface, herbs possess other chemical attributes. Among these are aromatic properties. Aromatherapy, as it has become known, makes use of the fragrant therapeutic values of herbs. Aromatherapists use oils or steams, which release volatile oils, during massage to affect the skin. Many health practitioners use these oils to treat physical conditions such as arthritis and chest congestion. Industry is adding herbal fragrances to air circulation systems in the workplace to inspire better humor and to increase productivity. A 1994 study in Japan showed that the use of peppermint oil in an air filtration system increased productivity and improved attitudes. We all know how certain smells can turn us "on" or "off". In fact, because of their chemical properties, herbal oils can stimulate or depress body and brain functions in their interpretation of a situation into an emotion or memory. But that's another subject.

When evaluating the choices for skin care, my utmost concern is using substances that support the skin's natural function to hold the body together and maintain the acid mantle. Skin naturally takes care of and protects itself; it fights bacteria and even turns dark or tans as a form of protection. (Tanning, or increased melanin, is a natural immune response to ultra-violet rays.) Skin strives to maintain balance, no matter what our environment, diet, or topical treatments do to disrupt it. For instance, if you apply a substance that is too alkaline, the skin will immediately begin working to restore its natural pH balance of 4.5 to 5.5. Many women notice that their make-up base changes color or disappears after a few hours. So they may apply another coat for the afternoon, perhaps another for the evening. In the meantime, the skin is struggling to keep up with the routine nature intended, that of protecting and cleansing through perspiration and oil production. Such action, on a daily basis, puts undue stress on the skin. This does not mean that you cannot occasionally apply something to your skin to stimulate a reaction such as increased cell regeneration. The operative word here is occasionally. Be sure you know the consequences of that application and how to follow up for maximum, safe results. For instance, burning the skin with acid can cause dryness, flaking, and redness. This reaction can be countered with an antiseptic and cell stimulant followed by an application of oil or other moisturizer.

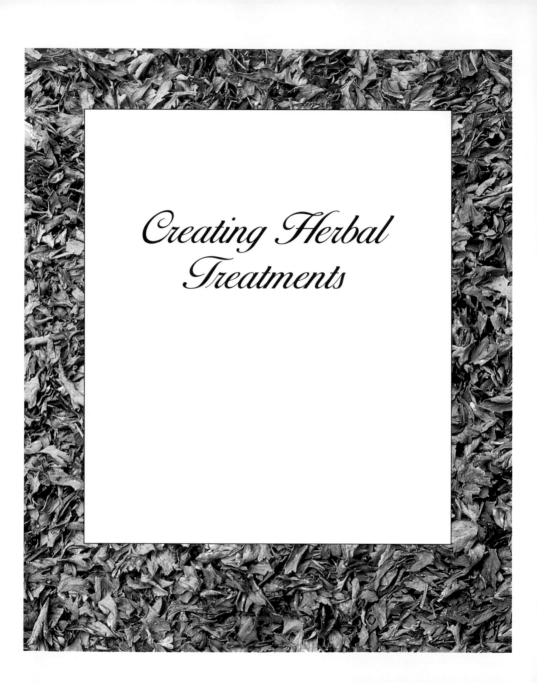

Creating Herbal Treatments

Herbs seem to be the safest and most effective choice for topical application. They are organic substances with known chemical constituents. With a little study, you can choose a single herb or simple combinations to achieve your goals.

It's easy. If you want to cleanse, use a saponic herb. To restore the acid mantle, which is affected by diet and environment, use an acidic herb with a pH of about 5 on a daily basis. For bacteria control, an astringent would help. But remember, after any application that is radical, one that burns the skin, has a very high or low pH, or is abrasive, follow up with a treatment to calm and restore balance. The goal is to help your skin do its job as effectively as possible; you don't want to sabotage the skin and make it expend energy undoing what you have done to it. That includes exposure to sun, smog, heat, dehydration (through perspiration or lack of water consumption), or even fat starvation. Let's look at some of the therapeutic properties of herbs.

Herb Classifications

Aromatic—These are the herbs whose prominent qualities are volatile oils. The oils have varied effects; analgesic for pain relief, antiseptic for slowing growth of bacteria, or phenolic for disinfection. Most are good for treating acne-prone skin or acid burn.
Examples—peppermint, cloves, fennel, ginger, lemongrass, and chamomile.

Astringent—These are usually acidic and have the ability to precipitate proteins, producing a protective coating that has a binding or tightening effect. Some astringents are also antifungal and are helpful for skin exposed to excessive humidity which can cause athlete's foot or other such conditions.
Examples—comfrey, golden seal, peppermint, mullein, and lavender.

Glycoside—These herbs contain one or more sugar acids which irritate the skin and cause rapid cell reproduction, expediting dead cell sloughing. Glycolic acids are commonly used in the cosmetics industry.
Examples—willow, red clover, rosehips, and strawberries (as well as most fruits).

Mucilaginous—These herbs are a good choice for masques for decongesting thereby cleaning deeply. They contain starches and are slippery. Their ability to store water makes them useful as hydrators or firming masques which constrict the skin, forcing pores to close. They also absorb toxins, such as smog and hydrocarbons.
Examples—marshmallow root, comfrey, dandelion, and kelp.

Saponic—Saponic herbs are used for cleansing. Herbs that contain saponins effect a foaming action and are often alkaline. They help other substances such as dirt, grease, and hydrocarbons dissolve or break down.
Examples—yucca, ginseng, and alfalfa.

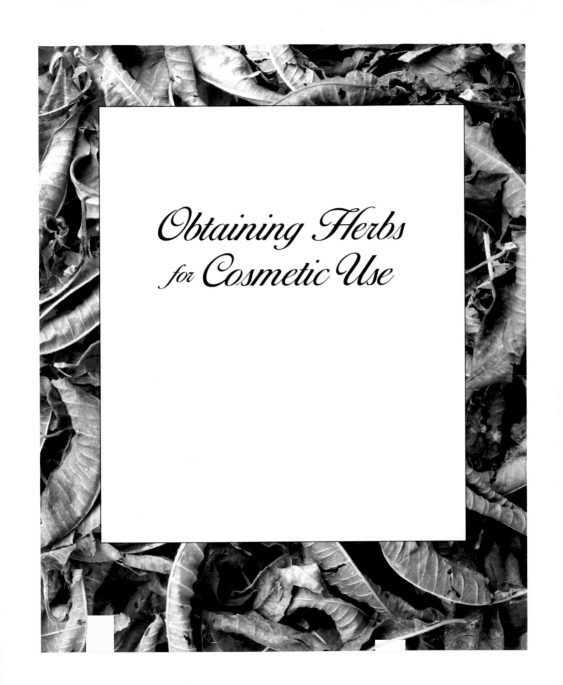

Obtaining Herbs
for Cosmetic Use

For maximum pleasure, once you have chosen one of the recipes that follow or invented a formula of your own, simply walk out to your garden, pick fresh, untreated herbs and prepare them for use. There are many texts available that can provide you with gardening basics, and most nurseries, garden centers, and even discount stores have a good, basic selection of herb plants. Check the recommended growing conditions and plant your herbs in the proper environment. My experience has been that most herbs grow well with reasonable neglect. After all, many herbs are considered weeds in some part of the world.

You can plant an elaborate herb garden or integrate herbs into your existing landscape. Make sure your plants will be accessible for picking and do not spray or otherwise treat them with poisons.

Condominium and apartment dwellers can also be successful herb gardeners; herbs grow in pots and window boxes quite happily, and many grow indoors or out.

If you don't have the time, space, or interest in growing your own herbs, you can find an ever-growing selection of fresh-cut herbs in the produce departments of many grocery stores. You may also purchase them dried from health food stores or by mail order. Most recipes require rehydration for use. It is very important that you use organic (pesticide free) herbs.

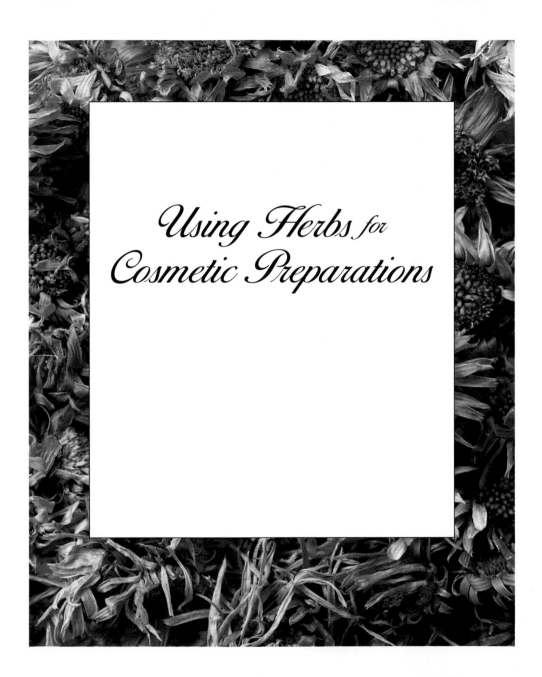

*Using Herbs for
Cosmetic Preparations*

There are many ways to use herbs; the following are the most common for cosmetic preparation.

Infusions—The weakest of preparations, infusions are good for hydrating. Using the leaves or flowers of the plant, steep them in simmering 200°F water as you would tea for about five minutes. Do not boil. Because of the runny, liquid nature of the mixture, you may soak some up with cheesecloth and apply the cloth to the skin. You may also seal infusions onto the skin by applying olive or safflower oil on top of them; then they may be removed with a warm washcloth. Depending on the herb you choose, an infusion may be used as a toner, an astringent, or a soother.

Decoctions—Use a decoction as you would an infusion, but when a more potent treatment is desired. Immerse the bark, roots, or seeds of a plant in water brought to a simmer. I like them to simmer for at least fifteen minutes and up to twenty-four hours. More concentrated than an infusion, it contains more volatile oils of the plant.

Macerations—Macerations, like decoctions, are concentrated, potent herbal fusions. Fill a sterilized jar with crushed herbs, dried or fresh. Cover with vegetable oil, cider vinegar, rubbing alcohol, or a grain alcohol such as vodka. Cover the jar and allow the mixture to stand for two weeks, shaking daily. Drain and strain the liquid into a sterilized bottle and use as desired. Oil macerations may be used for massage as lipophylic treatments; vinegars as toners, hair rinses, or additions to foot soaks; and alcohols as toners, astringents, antiseptics, and cleansers. Macerations will keep in the refrigerator for two months. Warm to room temperature before use.

Poultices—These draw out impurities from deep within the pores. Moisten herbs with hot water, about 200°F, allow them to cool enough to prevent burning, and wrap them in cheesecloth or muslin. Apply a poultice to the skin while still warm and remove when cool. Poultices can help greasy or acne-prone skin, and are invaluable for those who do mechanical work around heavy oils or who do a lot of food frying.

Masques—Masques are used to tighten the skin, stimulate circulation, and remove dead cells. Mix your chosen herb with a liquid such as water, milk, or aloe vera gel. You may also choose to add other substances such as clay, salt, or sugar. Masques are applied to the skin and left to dry; remove by gently wiping the skin with a water-dampened washcloth.

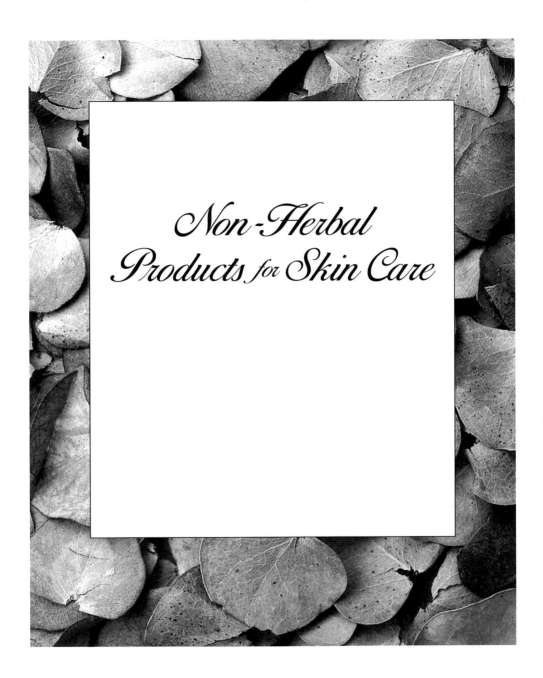

Non-Herbal Products for Skin Care

In addition to herbs, there are many other natural substances that are beneficial to the skin. They are used as carriers or as active ingredients in the formulas.

Abrasives—These are sand-like or granular substances that "scrub" the surface of the skin and remove dead cells. Abrasive treatments should not be used daily as they may cause irritation and begin a chain reaction of topical problems. I recommend using abrasives no more than twice weekly. Crushed fruit pits are commonly used commercially, with apricot being the most popular. However, I do not use or recommend apricot pits because they contain the chemical constituent cyanide, and massive doses could be harmful. I recommend crushed date pits as a scrub for removal of dead cells and impurities. Date oil is an antioxidant, and the points formed when crushing the pits are not as sharp as those of apricots. However, there is a danger in scrubbing with any crushed pits; tiny bits are sharp and can cut the skin. The resulting marred skin will feel rough and may prompt you to scrub again the next day, which would definitely not be a good idea. Some of my favorite abrasives are cane sugar (glycoside), powdered herbs such as parsley (salicylic acid), salt, some sands (silica), and nut powders, which have a lipophilic effect. Abrasives are best used with a carrier such as oil or water. The carrier allows smooth sloughing without damage to the lower layers of the skin.

Acids—Acids are usually used as toners, astringents, or peeling agents. Malac, tartaric, citric, and salycilic acids are found in parsley and chamomile as well as apples, grapes, and lemons. It is important to follow an alkaline cleansing treatment with an acidic one to bring the pH of the skin back to its normal state of between 4.5 and 5.5. Another acidic treatment is the "new" alpha hydroxy acid skin peel. The treatment is hardly new—Cleopatra's milk baths contained lactic acid, an alpha hydroxy acid, which removed the upper layer of skin to reveal smooth, new skin. Once you know the fruits and herbs that contain glycosides (sugar acids), you can create your own peels.

Note: When using acids, there is danger of burning the skin too deeply. Consult a cosmetic chemist or doctor before choosing your acid and the strength of it. I recommend that you start with an 8% alpha hydroxy level and raise that slightly each week if there is no swelling, broken skin, or sores. Do not exceed a level of 27%, that of pure lemon juice. Most products sold over-the-counter have a maximum of 12% glycolic or alpha hydroxy acid. So proceed with caution. Always do a test on a small patch of skin on the back of your hand before applying any treatment to any other part of your body, even if the treatment was recommended by a doctor.

Alkalies—Alkalies are usually used for cleansing, but they strip oils and moisture from the skin as well as impurities. That is why you may find that most soaps dry your skin. Soaps contain sodium hydroxide, commonly known as lye, and their pH range is usually above 8, more like 10, or about the same as many alkaline permanent wave solutions for the hair. This fact gave me second thoughts about using soap as a facial cleanser! If you use soap, be sure to follow the cleansing with an acid treatment to restore normal pH, and with a hydrophilic/lipophilic moisturizer.

Carriers—In most cases, these are lipophilic oils. Vegetable oils such as sunflower, wheat germ, and sesame have high levels of essential fatty acids which seal or hold the other substances on the skin. One of my favorite carriers is olive oil because of its acidic and antioxidant values. Wheat germ oil and is also a good antioxidant (although wheat germ itself oxidizes quickly). Vitamin A oil is found in fish or cod liver oil; it acts as a natural antibiotic and is good in formulas for blemished skin. Carrot oil is also rich in vit-

amin A. Evening primrose oil is commonly used cosmetically to reduce the appearance of wrinkles, but it is not one of my choices, as it is reported to affect estrogen levels when taken internally. While ingesting for skin treatment is not recommended, I avoid it topically, just in case. Avocado oil is rich in vitamins A and E. Use the whole avocado flesh and get protein and acids as well. Glycerin is smooth with a high hydrophilic factor. Since it has a low lipophilic factor, it should be used in conjunction with oils. Honey is cleansing and antibacterial. Milk is high in hydrophilic and lipophilic factors with the added benefits of vitamins and sugars.

Clays—These are usually used to draw out impurities through absorption. I remember Dad putting mud on our insect bites or bee stings to "draw out the poison". Clays are composed of silica, iron, magnesium, calcium, sodium, zinc, and other minerals. They help remove old sebum (oil) clogged in pores, hydrocarbon deposits from smog, old cosmetic wax buildup, contaminants from the workplace such as copier toner, and airborne oils through absorption, and they are also slightly abrasive. French rose clay tends to attract light oils. Green clay, also from France, has a high mineral content and attracts heavy clogging oils. It is good for oily or acne-prone skin. Bentonite is a white clay found in the midwestern United States. Its electromagnetic quality attracts oils and other particles. And, of course, there is still good old mud from your own backyard (be sure it is clean, that is, free of animal waste, pesticides, and lawn chemicals).

Proteins—Proteins are usually used for refining the surface of the skin by tightening wrinkles and closing pores. The word you will hear most from the commercial cosmetics world is collagen. Collagen is the protein complex produced in the germinative layers (dermis) of your skin. It forms the fibers that hold your skin up and give it support and form. Depletion of collagen through lack of vitamin C, alcohol consumption, smoking, and oxidation causes sagging and wrinkling. However, topical application has not proven to augment that collagen level. To the best of my knowledge, collagen production in the skin is directly related to vitamin C intake (vitamin C). Good proof of this is that the skin of smokers tends to wrinkle much more than that of nonsmokers; each cigarette depletes the body of 50 mg of vitamin C. Eating foods that are high in vitamin C will better feed the dermis and replenish collagen than the application of any cream. However, I do use proteins such as egg white and gelatin in masques; these help to tighten pores and refine small surface wrinkles. Protein masques are drying, so good follow-up with an astringent or toner and moisturizer is important.

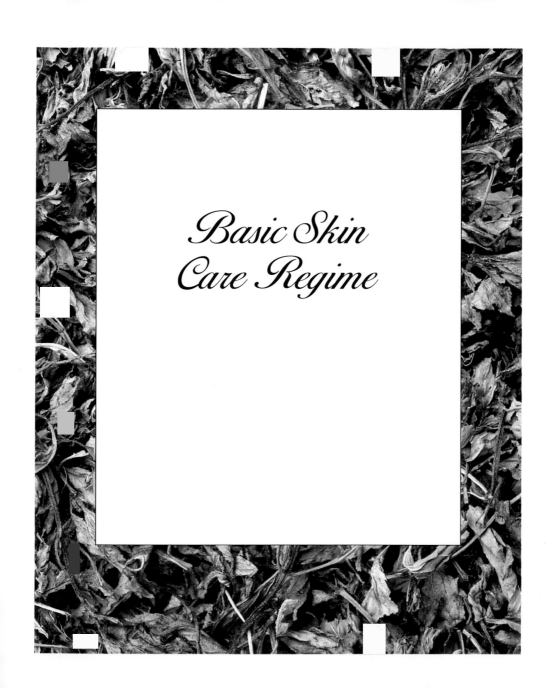

Basic Skin Care Regime

Before we begin, let me stress two important factors to remember in skin care:

1. Never put very hot or very cold water on the face. Extreme temperature will engorge or constrict capillaries too quickly. This can cause capillaries to break, resulting in the appearance of spider veins.

2. Never use petroleum products such as mineral oil, petrolatum, or microcrystalline waxes on the skin. They are occlusive, that is, they clog the pores and cause them to become enlarged.

Here are the basic steps to follow for healthy skin.

Cleanse to remove surface dirt, accumulated old oil, and daily pollutants.

Tone to restore skin's natural acid mantle.

Masque to reach impurities deep in the pores.

Protect from the elements, pollutants, and sun.

Hydro/Lipophilic replacement to rebalance moisture and oil in the skin.

In addition, specialized treatments may include:

Exfoliating by scrubbing with abrasives to remove dead cells.

Exfoliating with acids.

Refining with proteins.

Maximum healing or treatment masques to restore balance so the skin can function as nature intended.

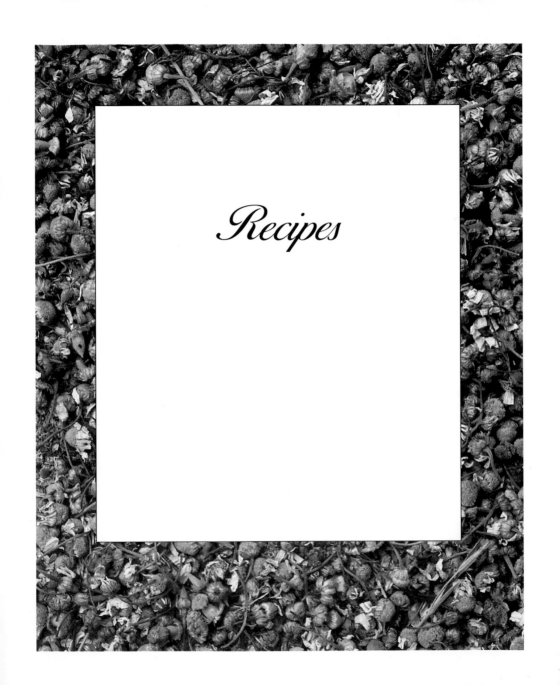

Recipes

SUPPLIES

Most of what you need is probably already in your kitchen.

- 1/2 cup to 1 quart hot/cold proof glass bowls
- Small and large whisks and spoons
- Wooden ice cream sticks (for stirring)
- Small electric food processor or chopper
- Small electric coffee cup warmer (a tiny hot plate)
- Various empty jars and lids, sanitized with boiling water
- Plastic ziplock sandwich bags

You may discover other helpful gadgets along the way. I like to devote a shelf or cupboard to my basic sanitized supplies so that I know they are ready when I am.

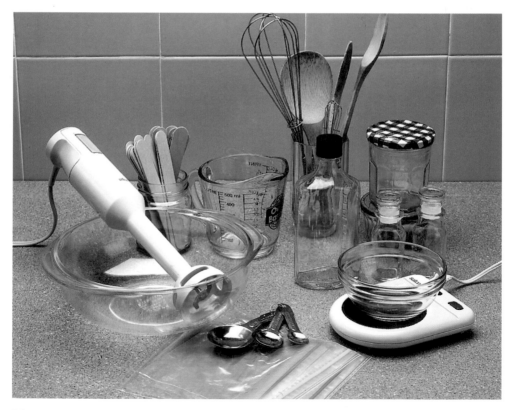

APPLICATION OF FORMULAS

I strongly advise that you use your own, clean fingers to apply formulas to your skin. While cotton balls and face brushes feel good, they may absorb some of the important constituents of the mixture. They might even have a negative effect. I once had a client who kept having an allergic reaction of eye irritation and swelling. The dilemma was that it was always worse after I gave her a facial treatment; and it didn't make sense. We started eliminating my formulas one by one. There was no change, and that was in some ways a relief. But still we were perplexed. Then one day during her treatment, I noticed that her hands were broken out. Oh no, it was spreading! When I asked what caused the rash on her hands, she replied, "Oh, I rode horses this weekend, and I'm allergic to them. I always break out when I ride." Further inquiry revealed that her expensive makeup brushes that she used after her facials were made of horse hair! Mystery solved. Moral: Use your own hands to apply formulas.

LET'S GET STARTED

These formulas are equally good for men and women. The first rule of skin treatment is **do not use any product on your skin that you already know you are sensitive to.** And I don't mean just topically; if you can't eat honey, don't put it on your face! I cannot stress this point too much. I had a client who failed to tell me of her allergy to cucumbers; she didn't think they would affect her skin. *Wrong!*

Rather than make a long list of herbs and their properties, I will explain their values with each recipe as they appear. You may wish to start a reference chart for these. It will be helpful in creating your own formulas.

Facial Cleansing Formulas

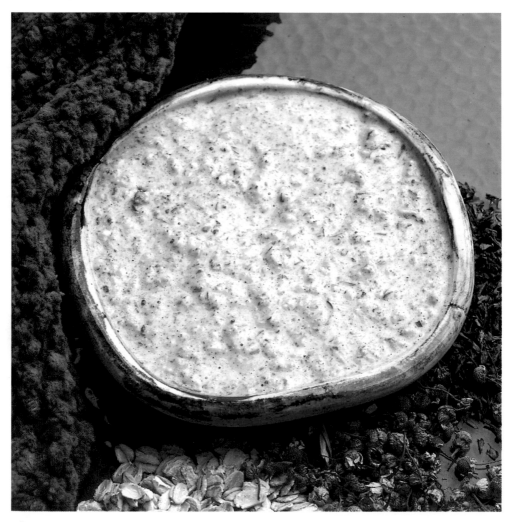

Cleansers should do just that, cleanse. Do not expect a cleanser to instill moisture or provide any other major treatment. It is important to follow a cleansing treatment with a toner that will restore the acid mantle of the face. Follow the toner with a moisturizer or oil.

Most of these cleansing formulas make enough for one or two applications unless otherwise indicated.

Cleanser for Normal Skin

This cleanser contains oats, which are saponic, and I have found that parsley and chamomile will thoroughly cleanse the grime of the week.

2 tablespoons oats
1 teaspoon parsley, fresh chopped or dried
1/4 teaspoon dried chamomile
1/4 cup hot water

Combine all ingredients and allow the oats to absorb the water and form a paste. Wet your face with tepid water, then apply the mixture. If the paste does not spread easily, add more water. You may remove this cleanser immediately with a washcloth dampened with tepid water or leave it to dry as a deep-cleaning masque. If you leave it to dry, moisten the mixture with a wet washcloth and wipe it off.

Sage and thyme are antiseptic and antibiotic in effect, and good for skin that is acne-prone or has large pores. Buttermilk enhances cleansing by breaking down dead skin cells, dirt, and other impurities on the surface of the skin, and its astringent action also makes it a good choice for skin with large pores because it will tighten or tone the tissue.

1/4 teaspoon sage, fresh or dried
1/4 teaspoon thyme, fresh or dried
1 tablespoon buttermilk

Combine all ingredients. Cover and allow to stand at least one hour at room temperature or overnight in the refrigerator for use the following day. Apply to the face with your fingertips and leave on for 3 to 5 minutes. Remove with a warm, damp washcloth. This formula may be used three times per week.

Cleanser for Dry Skin

This cleanser consists of honey, powdered milk, and yucca. Honey attracts moisture from the air and is good for peeling away dead cells. Powdered milk also enhances cleansing by breaking down dead skin cells, dirt, and other impurities on the surface of the skin. Yucca is a saponic herb, a natural cleanser with foaming qualities.

1 tablespoon honey
1 teaspoon powdered milk
1 teaspoon yucca, powdered
1 teaspoon warm water

Mix all ingredients let stand 10 minutes. Apply to a wet face with a lightly circular motion. Remove by rinsing with warm water, and follow with toner and non-petroleum moisturizer. This cleanser may be used up to twice per week.

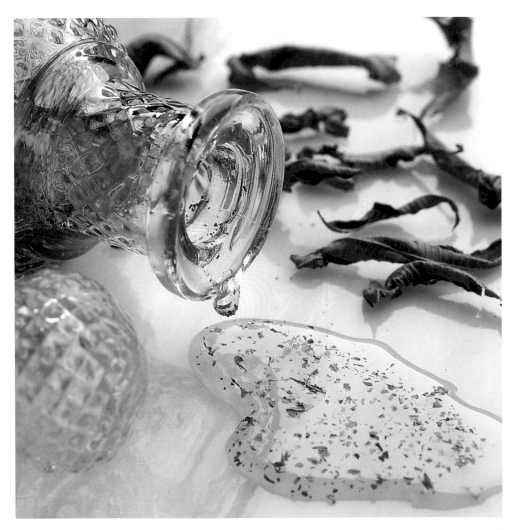

Toners restore acidity to the skin
after cleansing. They are astringent and
contain tannins that have a tightening effect,
which make them helpful for reducing large
pores. They are also antibacterial agents.
Toners can have a drying effect on the skin
and should always be followed with a
non-petroleum moisturizer or oil.

Toner for Normal Skin

Apple cider vinegar is a form of acetic acid which restores acid pH. Usually with a pH of 2, the vinegar is too strong to use alone; water must be added to bring the pH up to 4 or 5, otherwise it can cause irritation from acid burn. Lemon verbena contains volatile oils that are astringent.

1 teaspoon apple cider vinegar
2 tablespoons water
1/4 teaspoon lemon verbena, dried and crushed

Combine all ingredients and let stand 3 to 5 minutes or overnight. After cleansing your face, use your fingers and a wiping motion to apply the toner. As soon as it dries, remove it with a tepid wet washcloth. Apply moisturizer while your skin is still damp.

This toner should be used no more than three times per week. It may be refrigerated in a sterilized bottle for one week.

Toner for Oily Skin

This toner can also be used as a refresher after exercise.

Warning: This formula is not good for sensitive skin with weak capillaries; it may be an irritant and cause capillaries to break. Peppermint has refreshing antibacterial volatile oils. Lemon juice is acidic with some sugars and has antibacterial properties.

1/4 teaspoon peppermint, dried or fresh and crushed
1/4 teaspoon sage, dried or fresh and crushed
1 teaspoon lemon juice, fresh, not bottled
2 tablespoons water

Mix all ingredients together and let stand at least 5 minutes to overnight to release the volatile oils. Apply with your fingers to a clean face. As soon as the mixture has dried, remove gently with a washcloth wet with tepid water. Your face may be red from the acid and volatile oils, but the redness should disappear within a few hours. Use no more than once a week.

Toner for Dry Skin

Very simple but effective, witch hazel is astringent. Lavender is antibacterial and promotes cell reproduction. Rosehips contain vitamin C or ascorbic acid and sugars.

1 tablespoon witch hazel
1/2 teaspoon lavender, fresh or dried
1/4 teaspoon rosehips, dried and crushed or powdered

Combine ingredients and allow to stand at least one day. Apply to clean face with fingertips. This toner may be removed with a washcloth wet with tepid water or left on the skin. If you leave it on, apply moisturizer before the toner dries.

Hydrating Formulas

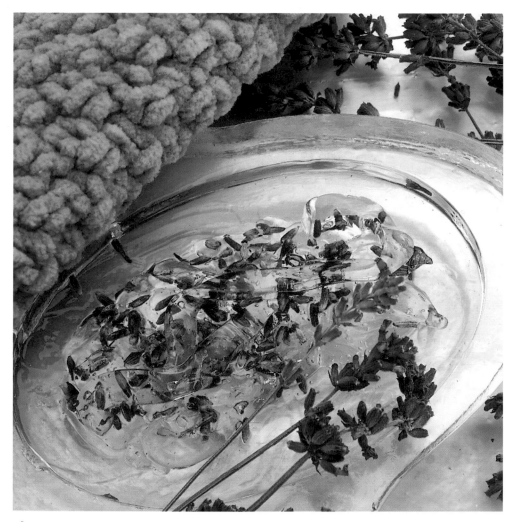

Hydrating formulas are used to introduce moisture to the skin. Because they are not combined with any oil or lipophilic ingredient, it is extremely important to follow treatment with a lipophilic or oil product. You may add a small amount of your favorite oil to these recipes, making them hydro/lipophilic in nature.

I choose not to include oils as they might interfere with the skin's ability to absorb the valuable constituents of the herbs.

I prefer to use the follow-up oil method.

Rosewater and glycerin are old time favorites, and rightly so. Glycerin is softening because it is soluble with water. The volatile oils in rosewater are soothing, both in fragrance and in action. It will not irritate the skin or overstimulate circulation. Food grade rosewater can usually be found in a liquor store; it is an old fashioned ingredient in some mixed drinks. Rosehips contain acids and vitamin C which smooth the skin. In this strength, they are astringent, or tightening.

1/2 tablespoon glycerin
1/2 tablespoon rosewater
1/4 teaspoon rosehips, ground

Mix all ingredients and allow to stand at least 5 minutes. Apply with fingers to a clean, wet face. You may leave the solution on for up to 15 minutes. I like to spray distilled water over my face while the solution is on and massage it in before removing with a washcloth dampened with cool water.

A Drink for Your Face

Aloe vera gel has long been revered for its healing abilities and it retains moisture. Lavender has antiseptic volatile oils. I use distilled water in this recipe because it doesn't contain the minerals that tap water does. (Most of the other recipes are more acidic and buffer the minerals.)

1/2 tablespoon aloe gel
1 tablespoon lavender blossoms, crushed
1/2 tablespoon distilled water

Combine all ingredients and allow to stand 1/2 to 24 hours. Apply to a clean face and leave on for 1/2 hour. If the mixture has dried, rewet with water and remove with a washcloth. Follow this treatment with a non-petroleum moisturizer or olive oil.

CONDITIONING FORMULAS

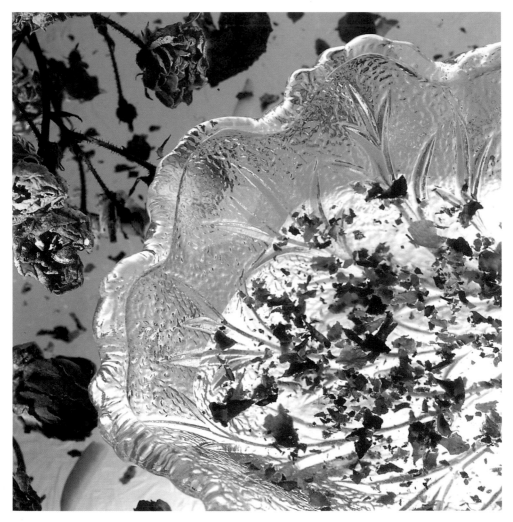

Lipophilic or conditioning formulas help your skin retain the moisture that you apply as well as that you drink. The formulas should be left on for at least 30 minutes, up to a few hours. They make very good night treatments, or you may apply them before settling in with a good book or your favorite music. Apply after a thorough cleansing and toning.

Sunflower and sesame oils are rich but not occlusive or smothering. They are filled with nutrients and essential fatty acids that smooth your skin. Rose petals are soothing and contain a small amount of vitamin C; ascorbic acid will smooth and tone the skin. Crushed almonds are rich with vitamins and just abrasive enough to be smoothing. This is a great treatment for that special afternoon or evening you have to yourself. Take a bath with it on—the steam will make it work better!

1 teaspoon sunflower oil
1 teaspoon rose petals, crushed
1 teaspoon sesame oil
1/2 teaspoon almond, powdered or crushed

Mix the ingredients together and apply to a water-moistened, cleaned, and toned face. Relax at least a half hour, preferably more. Spray your face occasionally with distilled water and massage. This solution may be left on all night, or you may remove it with a washcloth dampened with warm water. **Warning:** Do not wear this treatment in the sun! The mixture attracts and intensifies ultra violet rays which cause sunburn.

After the Ball

Olive oil is acidic and acts as a preservative when used on foods. On skin, it helps to slow oxidation or aging. Calendula petals, often used in herbal healing mixtures for wounds, soften the skin and are antiseptic and antifungal. Violet flowers have deliciously scented volatile oils and I find it to be softening. Orange blossoms, like the violet, have soothing, fragrant volatile oils. Deliciously relaxing "after the ball" or a wonderful evening, this treatment is equally satisfying during the day when you can just relax.

1 tablespoon olive oil
1 / 2 teaspoon calendula petals, dried and crushed
1 teaspoon violet flowers, fresh or dried
1 teaspoon orange blossoms, fresh or dried

Place all ingredients in a small, heat-proof glass bowl. Warm on coffee cup warmer or over very low heat on the stove. Allow the mixture to cool to a comfortable temperature and massage it on a cleaned, toned, and water-moistened face. Leave it on for at least 30 minutes or for hours longer if desired. This makes a nice night oil and may be used 3 to 4 times per week on dry skin or twice monthly on oily skin. **Warning:** Do not wear this treatment in the sun! The mixture attracts and intensifies ultra violet rays which cause sunburn.

Hydro-/Lipophilic Treatments

These formulas provide both oil and water to the skin. Enjoy the softness that these treatments provide. They feel wonderful on stressed or polluted skin. Cleanse well and tone before application.

The whole milk called for in this recipe contains both fat and water with vitamins and sugars. Linden flowers are calming. Mullein flowers have saponins, volatile oils, and glycosides. Safflower oil contains vitamin A and has a slight anti-inflammatory effect.

1½ tablespoons whole milk
1/2 teaspoon linden flowers, dried and crushed
1/2 teaspoon mullein flowers, fresh or dried and crushed
1/2 teaspoon safflower oil

Combine all ingredients allow to stand 30 minutes. Apply to clean and toned skin. Leave on for at least 12 minutes to ensure the release of the oils. Remove with a washcloth dampened with warm water. Follow with the toner for dry skin and a light moisturizer. You may use this one twice a week. (More frequent use may cause congestion in the pores.)

Sheared Delight

This recipe uses lanolin oil. Lanolin oil is the most compatible with human skin oil in a molecular sense. Unfortunately, lanolin is very dirty when extracted from sheared wool. Because some techniques used for cleaning lanolin require solvents that can cause allergic reactions in many people, you may hear many dermatologists advise against its use. But a pure, filtered, and pasteurized lanolin should pose no problems. The lavender has an antibacterial effect. Elder flowers contain glycosides for smoothing; they irritate and loosen dead cells. The coconut milk is rich in fat as well as water.

1/2 tablespoon lanolin oil
1/2 teaspoon lavender flowers, fresh or dried and crushed
1/4 teaspoon elder flowers, dried and crushed
1/2 tablespoon coconut milk

Combine all ingredients in small, heat-proof glass bowl. Heat on coffee cup warmer, or on a stove top burner set to very low, until just warm and stir until blended. Do not allow to boil or steam. Boiling or steaming will change the chemistry of the mixture and it will become too acidic. Allow to cool to a temperature that you can comfortably apply to the skin. Apply the mixture to the face and leave on for 15 minutes. Remove with a washcloth dampened with warm water.

WHIPPED CREAM DELIGHTS

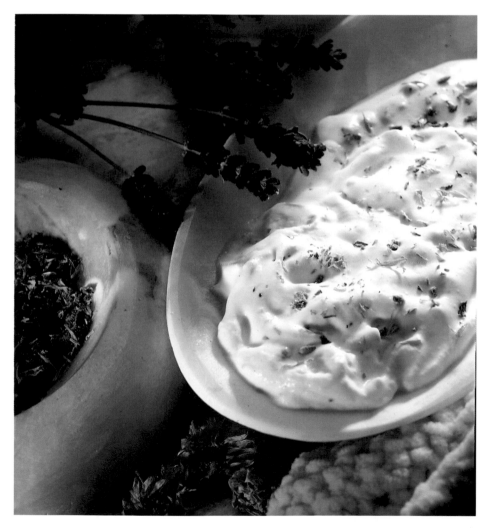

Somewhat too rich to eat,
the fats, moisture, sugars, and enzymes
in whipped cream can work wonders in
smoothing and enriching the skin.
These recipes may be prepared with a food
processor or whipped by hand.
Whipping cream turns to butter quickly.
If this happens, you may use the mixture
anyway; it will just be a bit messier and
a bit more challenging to apply.

Rose petals contain fragrant and soothing volatile oils, and lavender has both antibacterial and volatile oil qualities. Calendula is important here for its softening effects.

1/4 cup whipping cream
1/2 teaspoon rose petals, fresh or dried
1/2 teaspoon lavender flowers, fresh or dried
1/2 teaspoon calendula petals, dried

Combine all ingredients in a food processor or bowl and whip until stiff peaks form. Apply the creamy mixture to your face and/or to dry skin on other parts of the body. Leave the mixture on for at least 10 minutes, then remove with a washcloth dampened with warm water. Follow with a witch hazel toner and apply a light, non-petroleum moisturizer. You may use this treatment 3 times per week on very dry skin, once every 10 days for oilier skin.

Italian Moon Mist

This mixture calls for a lovely combination of Mediterranean herbs and oils. Avocado is rich in essential fatty acids and vitamins A and E. The olive oil in this preparation not only supplies fats, but also provides antioxidant action—notice that if you have some left over, the avocado does not turn black as soon as normal. Chamomile is antibacterial.

1/4 cup whipping cream
1 tablespoon avocado, the real thing, not oil
1 teaspoon olive oil
1 teaspoon chamomile, dried

Combine all ingredients in a food processor or bowl and whip until stiff peaks form. Apply to the skin and leave on for at least 10 minutes. Remove with a washcloth dampened with warm water. If it is night time, you need not follow with anything. The residue should be adequate night protection from dehydration. This one is ever, ever so rich. Like an Italian meal and romantic evening in Venezia.

Oats are saponic and soften the skin. Calendula is softening and healing. Sunflower oil is rich in vitamin A which is a natural antibiotic and contains essential fatty acid. Rosewater is relaxingly fragrant and supplies volatile oils. This masque leaves the skin feeling as fresh as a country day in spring.

1/4 cup whipping cream
1 teaspoon calendula petals, fresh or dried
1 teaspoon sunflower oil
1 tablespoon rosewater (food grade)

Combine all ingredients and allow to stand for 3 minutes. Whip in processor or by hand until stiff peaks or thick paste form. Add more cream if the mixture is too dry to whip. Apply to water-moistened skin and leave on for 10 minutes. Remove the mixture with a washcloth dampened with warm water and follow with toner and moisturizer. Sorry, this one is a bit messy, but oh, so worth it!

SPECIAL TREATMENTS

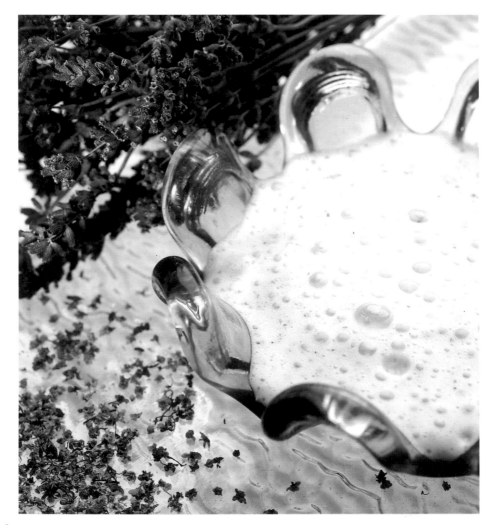

Clean and Tidy

This formula is especially good for oily or acne-prone skin. Parsley, red clover, and lavender will cleanse and tone the skin.

1/8 teaspoon parsley, dried and crushed
1/8 teaspoon red clover, dried and crushed or powdered
1/2 teaspoon lavender blossoms, fresh or dried and crushed
1½ tablespoons hot water

Combine all ingredients and allow to stand for 3 minutes. Wet the face with water, then wash with the mixture. Be sure not to be too abrasive to avoid scratching the epidermis. Just spread the mixture around. Because of the acids, this treatment may cause a slight burning sensation but that is what is giving you the benefit. Do not use this one on skin that is sensitive or gets broken capillaries easily.

Margarine is hydrogenated fats. While it may not be good in your diet, it is a wonderful hydro-/lipophilic formula for the surface of your skin. Lavender and calendula have volatile oils. Calendula is also antifungal, and lavender is a relaxant. Any leftovers of this formula may be refrigerated in an airtight container for one week, or rolled up in wax or plastic wrap and frozen for one month. If frozen, cut off small portions as you need them. *Hint:* Use the cheapest store brand of margarine. These usually contain more than one kind of oil and have more water in them than most brand names. Dried herbs are better than fresh here, especially if you are going to save any of the mixture; adding too much moisture could upset the chemical balance, possibly promoting fermentation.

1/4 cup margarine
2 teaspoons lavender flowers, dried and crushed
2 teaspoons calendula petals, dried and crushed

Combine all ingredients in a small, glass heat-proof bowl. Melt on a coffee cup warmer or on a stovetop burner set to very low. Allow the mixture to cool until it is solid. Apply to water-moistened skin with the fingertips and leave on for 5 minutes. Remove with a washcloth dampened with warm water. Follow with a toner and oil or non-petroleum moisturizer. This formula is good to use on rough knees, elbows, and heels. Save remaining mixture as mentioned above. Use on the face no more than 2 times per week, daily if desired on knees, elbows, and heels. Can you believe it's not butter?

Help for the Pore

The egg white in this mixture contains proteins that bond and cause a tightening effect. Cornstarch is also tightening and absorbent. Lavender is antiseptic, and elder flowers will soften dead skin cells that will be picked up by the cornstarch.

1 egg white
1/4 teaspoon cornstarch
1/2 teaspoon lavender flowers, fresh or dried
1/2 teaspoon elder flowers

Combine all ingredients and whisk until foamy or stiff. Allow to stand 3 minutes, then apply to a clean face. Allow the mixture to dry on the skin. (It will feel very tight.) Remove with a washcloth wet with cold water by laying the washcloth over the face and leaving it long enough to soften the masque, then remove gently. Follow the treatment with toner and a non-petroleum moisturizer. Because this masque has a drying effect, the moisturizer is a must. You will love the smooth look this gives your face! Because this treatment is somewhat drying, use it only once or twice per week. If you choose to use this treatment regularly, I recommend using a heavier hydro/lipophilic replacement masque at least one other day of that week to rehydrate the skin. *Hint:* If your skin is very dry, use the whole egg (the yolk contains fats and essential fatty acids) and leave out the cornstarch.

MASQUES

Use masques for deep cleaning of the pores. Masques will also tighten the skin, stimulate circulation, and remove dead cells.

Clarifying Mineral Masque

Use this masque on blemished or oily skin. The green clay will absorb excessive heavy oils. The sage and lavender are antiseptic and resist the growth of acne-producing bacteria.

1 tablespoon green clay
1/2 teaspoon sage, ground
1 teaspoon lavender flowers, fresh or dried, crushed
1 1/2 tablespoons water

Combine all ingredients. Apply to a clean face and allow to dry. Remove with a washcloth wet with cool water. Lay the wet cloth over the face to soften masque, then remove gently. Follow with a non-petroleum moisturizer, as this masque is drying and the clay absorbs precious natural skin oils. This may be used once a week.

Rosy Clear

This treatment with help to clarify or decongest the top layer of drier skin. Rose clay is not as absorbent as green clay, thus making it more desirable for use on dry skin. Glycerin keeps the formula from totally absorbing the surface oils. Lavender is healing and antiseptic.

1 tablespoon rose clay
1 / 2 tablespoon glycerin
1 teaspoon lavender flowers, fresh or dried, crushed

Combine all ingredients to make a paste. Apply to a clean face and leave on for 3 to 5 minutes. Remove by rinsing with tepid water.

BATH TREATMENTS

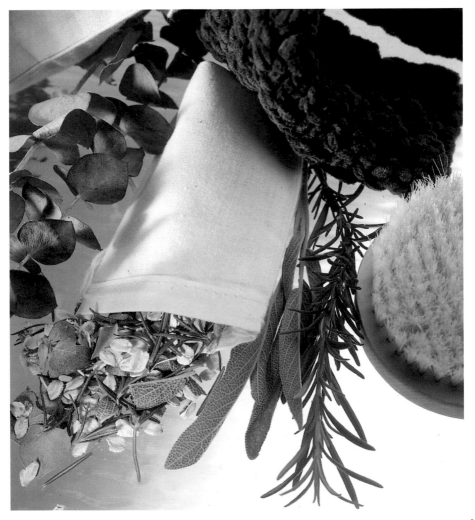

Bath bags are made by placing ingredients
into a piece of muslin or a handkerchief,
then securing them by tying the corners
together or tying with a ribbon or string.
Place the bag in the tub while you're filling
it with water. Acting like a giant tea bag,
it turns your bath into an herbal tea.
You may then use the soaked bag to scrub
and cleanse the surface of the skin.
If you prefer showers, take the bag of herbs
into the shower with you, soak it,
then use it like a wash cloth.

Calm and Clean

This is great for when you wish to relax. Lemon balm and orange blossoms will soothe the nervous system and skin surface. Violet leaves will soften and cleanse the skin. Oats are saponic and contain plenty of proteins and vitamins.

1 tablespoon lemon balm, fresh or dried
1 teaspoon orange blossoms
1 tablespoon violet leaves, fresh from your yard if they're not sprayed, or dried
1/4 cup rolled oats

Place all ingredients in a muslin bag and put the bag in the tub as you fill it with water.

When you've worked all day and still have a meeting to attend at night, you may feel the need for a pick-me-up. This treatment will give you a boost of energy. Because it is so stimulating, do not use this just before going to bed or trying to relax. Rosemary and sage are stimulating, and the volatile oils in eucalyptus are refreshing. The saponic oats fill the cleansing role.

1 tablespoon rosemary, fresh or dried
1 teaspoon sage, fresh or dried
1/2 tablespoon eucalyptus leaves, fresh or dried
1/4 cup oats

Place all ingredients in a muslin bag and put the bag in the tub as you fill it with water.

Post-Exercise Muscle Saver

Juniper berries are said to be antirheumatic and peppermint and spearmint contain volatile oils that are relaxing. Lavender is not only antiseptic, but is also a relaxant. People with arthritis will enjoy this bath.

1 teaspoon juniper berries
2 tablespoons peppermint, fresh or dried
2 tablespoons spearmint, fresh or dried
2 tablespoons lavender flowers and leaves, fresh or dried

Place all ingredients in a muslin bag and put the bag in the tub as you fill it with water.

AFTER BATH OILS

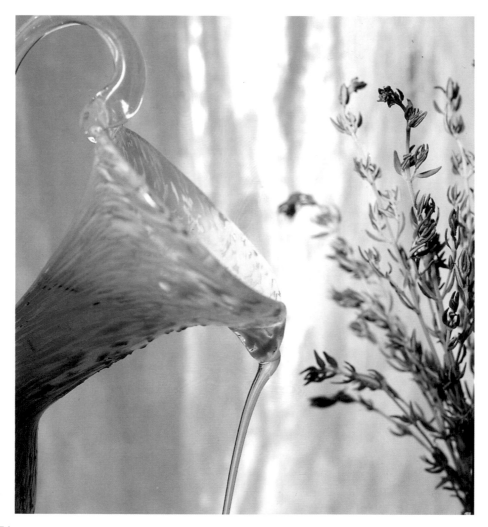

To condition the skin after a bath or shower, massage these oils onto your skin while it is still wet, then blot the skin dry with an old towel (there will be an oily residue left on the towel).

Your skin will feel silky smooth because you are providing it with the essential hydro and lipophilic factors. To release volatile oils, bruise herbs first by crushing them in your hand or in a plastic bag.

Sunflower oil is rich in vitamin A, a natural antibiotic with antioxidant properties. Lemon balm and rose petals contain relaxing volatile oils.

1/2 cup sunflower oil
1 tablespoon lemon balm, fresh
2 tablespoons rose petals, fresh

Combine all ingredients in a sanitized bottle. Allow to stand about a week to ensure release of the oils; they may then be stored in the refrigerator for up to three months. Use as needed for dry skin.

Ancient Energy

Sesame oil, although pungent, is very rich in vitamins A and E. The tannins in rosemary and thyme are purifying and astringent.

1/2 cup sesame oil
1 teaspoon rosemary, fresh
1 teaspoon thyme, fresh

Combine all ingredients in a sanitized bottle. Allow to stand about a week to ensure release of the oils; they may then be stored in the refrigerator for up to three months. Use as needed for dry skin.

Use extra virgin, Italian olive oil for its purity and acidity. The volatile oils in lemon verbena and mullein are both soothing and softening.

1/2 cup olive oil
1 teaspoon lemon verbena, fresh or dried
2 teaspoons mullein flowers, fresh or dried

Combine all ingredients in a sanitized bottle. Allow to stand about a week to ensure release of the oils; they may then be stored in the refrigerator for up to three months. Use as needed for dry skin.

Bath Vinegars

Vinegar is great for city water, which is very alkaline. Adding vinegar to your bath lowers the pH of the water, making it less harsh on the skin. The addition of therapeutic herbs is a wonderful bonus to your skin. I choose apple cider vinegar for the fruit acid. When you discover a recipe you particularly like, make it by the gallon. Pretty bottles of these and the oils make wonderful gifts.

Rosemary is stimulanting and astringent.

1 cup apple cider vinegar
2 tablespoons rosemary, dried or fresh

Combine ingredients in a sanitized bottle and set in a sunny place for a week, or heat the vinegar (do not boil) and then pour it over the herbs into the bottle. This recipe is for one treatment, making about one cup for one bath. For use in the shower, cleanse your body and then apply a small amount to a washcloth and wash with it. You could also strain it and apply it through a spray bottle. Do rinse after use.

Rosebuds and rosehips are both good sources of Vitamin C, and their volatile oils are relaxing.

1 cup apple cider vinegar
4 rose buds, fresh
2 teaspoons rosehips, dried and ground

Combine ingredients in a sanitized bottle and set in a sunny place for a week, or heat the vinegar (do not boil) and then pour it over the herbs into the bottle. This recipe is for one treatment, making about one cup for one bath. For use in the shower, cleanse your body and then apply a small amount to a washcloth and wash with it. You could also strain it and apply it through a spray bottle. Do rinse after use

Exertion Elixir

Eucalyptus and juniper have refreshing volatile oils.

1 cup apple cider vinegar
1½ teaspoon juniper berries, fresh or dried
1 tablespoon eucalyptus leaves, fresh or dried, crushed

   Combine ingredients in a sanitized bottle and set in a sunny place for a week, or heat the vinegar (do not boil) and then pour it over the herbs into the bottle. This recipe is for one treatment, making about one cup for one bath. For use in the shower, cleanse your body and then apply a small amount to a washcloth and wash with it. You could also strain it and apply it through a spray bottle. Do rinse after use

MASQUES FOR THE HANDS

Our hands are probably the most used
and abused parts of our bodies.
Treating them with cleansing and soothing
masques can reduce the outward signs
of stress and aging.

Spots Away

Oats are saponic and cleanse and soften the skin. Lemon juice contains citric acids which has a lightening or bleaching effect on age spots and freckles by peeling off outer layers of the epidermis. Calendula and honey are softening and healing.

2 tablespoons oats
2 teaspoons lemon juice, fresh
1 teaspoon calendula petals, fresh or dried
1 tablespoon honey
3 tablespoons warm water

Combine all ingredients in a chopper or grinder and work into a paste. Apply to clean, wet hands, and up the forearms to the elbows, if you like. Leave on for 5 minutes. Remove with tepid water and follow with a non-petroleum hand moisturizing lotion. You may use this treatment 3 times per week. You'll love it!

Olive oil, glycerin, and mullein flowers are all softening. The vinegar helps the skin to retain some of the softening agents and allows ingredients to be absorbed into the uppermost layers.

2 tablespoons extra-virgin olive oil
1 teaspoon mullein flowers, fresh or dried, crushed
1 teaspoon apple cider vinegar
2 teaspoons glycerin

Combine all ingredients, blend, and let stand for 10 minutes. Apply to clean skin and leave on for 15 minutes. For maximum softening, wrap the hands with warm, wet towels for the 15 minutes, then wipe off.

TREATMENTS FOR THE FEET

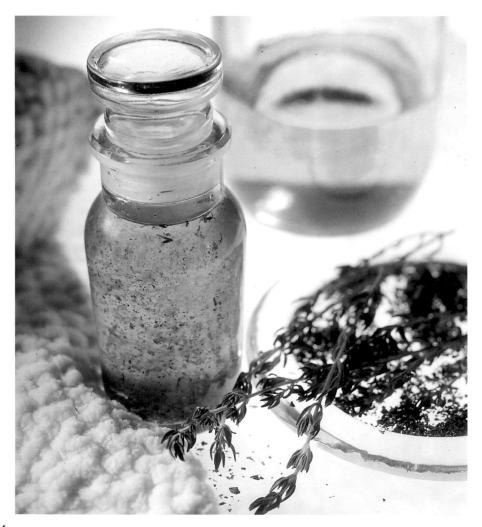

Foot Soak

The water in this foot soak should be as warm as is comfortable without scalding. Burdock root is softening and lavender is relaxing and antiseptic.

3 gallons warm water
1 cup apple cider vinegar
1 tablespoon burdock root
1 tablespoon lavender flowers, fresh or dried

Combine ingredients in a tub or bucket large enough in which to immerse your feet. For happy feet, soak them for 20 minutes.

Console Your Feet Massage Oil

I use olive oil in this formula for its lipophilic properties and its acidity. Thyme and marjoram are soothing, antiseptic, and help control odor by reducing bacteria. Use this after soaking or cleaning feet.

1/2 cup olive oil
1 teaspoon thyme, fresh or dried
1 teaspoon marjoram, fresh or dried

To release volatile oils, bruise herbs first by crushing them in your hand or in a plastic bag. Combine all ingredients in a sanitized bottle. Allow to stand about a week to ensure the release of volatile oils; you may then store the oil in the refrigerator for up to three months. Use as desired by massaging the oil onto your skin while it is still wet, then blotting it dry with an old towel (there will be an oily residue left on the towel).

TREATMENTS FOR THE HAIR

Now that we know how to
take care of our skin, let's put our best hair
forward as well!

Vinegar Hair Rinses

One-half cup of vinegar with one-half cup of water is what my mother always used on our hair. I now know that the acid rinse keeps the hair healthy and clean from residues, be they from hair spray, gel, or smog. Add certain herbs and you have a treatment.

Add to one-half cup vinegar and one-half cup water:

2 teaspoons chamomile for blonde hair.
Note: *Chamomile is used to dye yarn yellow, so do a test strand first.*

2 teaspoons sage for dark or oily hair.

Scalp Massage Oil and Hair Treatment

This mixture restores shine to the hair while acting as an antiseptic for dandruff.

1/4 cup olive oil
1 teaspoon sage, fresh or dried
1 teaspoon rosemary, fresh or dried

On clean wet scalp, part the hair in rows every inch and massage oil on. The oil may be combed through the hair and covered with a warm to hot wet towel for 5 minutes. The heat opens the cuticles so that the mixture can get into the hair shafts. Wash out with a mild shampoo.

BIBLIOGRAPHY

Balch, James F. *Prescription for Nutritional Healing.* Garden City Park, NY: Avery Publishing Group, Inc., 1990.

Barlow, Max G. *From the Shepherd's Purse.* Pocatello, ID: Spice West Publications, 1990.

Maine, Sandy. *The Soap Book.* Loveland, CO: Interweave Press, 1995.

Ody, Penelope. *The Complete Medicinal Herbal.* New York: Dorling Kindersley, 1993.

Pedersen, Mark. *Nutritional Herbology.* Warsaw, IN: Wendell W. Whitman Company, 1994.

Rothenberg, Mikel A. and Charles F. Chapman. *Dictionary of Medical Terms for the Nonmedical Person.* Hauppage, NY: Barron's, 1994.

Schlossberg, Leon. *Human Functional Anatomy, Third Edition.* Baltimore: Johns Hopkins Press, 1986.

Winter, Ruth. *A Consumer's Dictionary of Cosmetic Ingredients.* New York: Crown Publishers, Inc., 1984.

METRIC CONVERSIONS

1/8 teaspoon	0.5 ml
1/4 teaspoon	1 ml
1/2 teaspoon	2 ml
1 teaspoon	5 ml
1/2 tablespoon	7 ml
1 tablespoon	15 ml
1½ tablespoons	22 ml
2 tablespoons	30 ml
3 tablespoons	45 ml
1/4 cup	60 ml
1/2 cup	120 ml
1 cup	240 ml
1 gallon	3.75 liters

INDEX

95